# Herbal Medicine: Proven Alternative Homemade Remedies to Heal Without Pills

Table of Contents

## Introduction

Home remedies prove helpful to deal with lots of common and complex ailment. Luckily, there are numerous herbs that can be used to treat a number of ailments. Hiccups may be the most annoying and the funniest ailments.

Although these hiccups are not life threatening, they can still be annoying and cause discomfort. Hiccups usually result from many involuntary contractions of your diaphragm, which are the muscle between your abdomen and chest. Hiccups may be caused by misfired message from your brain that may get stuck in a continuously occurring loop.

The cure for hiccups is to swallow a teaspoon full of sugar, or you can even gargle with ice water for around 30 seconds. Hagen, a famous physician, says that both the tricks probably do send up a signal to your brain that may disrupt the message loop, which would allow your diaphragm to relax.

However, if your hiccups last for more than 48 hours or become severe that it is hard to eat or breathe, then you should contact a doctor. In rare cases, hiccups can be a symptom of brain injury, a stroke or even multiple sclerosis.

The cure for minor injuries is to place the small-burned area under running cold water for several minutes until all the pain has subsidies. This would also help to reduce the swelling. Then you should apply a thin layer of lotion that contains Aloe Vera a particular segment of an aloe leaf that is into cut lengthwise, which should be directly on the burn.

However, use takes caution when applying lotion to the potentially infected as it can seal in the infection and prevent proper healing. Hence, great care should be taken when healing with burns.

Congestion in chest and sneezing could result from a cold caused by some viral infection that may appear in your upper respiratory tract. The cure for cold and flu is simple that can be easily followed at home.  A bowl of chicken soup is the best remedy to fight cold and flu.

Even onion and garlic stock in the broth have anti-inflammatory, and the steam of these herbs helps clear up congestion. Chicken broth may also contain some enzymes that may have an anti-microbial effect. It is necessary for everyone to try healing with chicken soup recipe to banish your cold.

The cure eczema all you need to do is add a sprinkle of baking soda or even some uncooked oats to warm bath for skin-soothing effect. If that area becomes infected, then your doctor may recommend adding up a capful of bleach to your bath to get some relief.

The reason to this is that bleach kills any skin-irritating bacteria. You should make sure that you spend only five to 10 minutes in the tub and don't submerge your head in it. The emergency case that may require you to call your doctor is if you are too itchy to sleep, and you suspect that your skin is infected or your condition doesn't improve within a few days of treatment.

# Chapter 1 – Important Herbal Plants for Many Ailments

There are some important herbal plants that prove helpful for the treatment of various ailments. These plants are as under:

## Aloe Vera

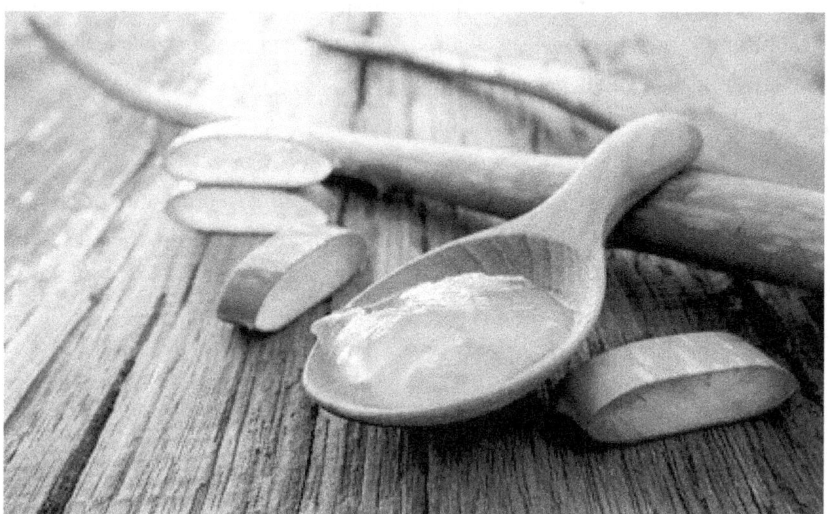

Aloe Vera is a natural anti-inflammatory agent, which tremendously has antibacterial elements in it as well. Aloe Vera has many different medicinal and other healing properties apart from cooling the body temperature and increasing its immunity.

Aloe gel is extracted from Aloe Vera from the aloe plant that can be used for treating several internal infections such as bacterial skin infections or vaginal and urinary tract infections. Aloe gel can always be applied directly to the area that is affected and also a quarter cup of juice that is consumed as well for treating the bacterial skin infections.

The anti-inflammatory and antibacterial properties of Aloe Vera are considered good to treat some bacterial infection naturally. Moreover, Aloe Vera also has healing and medicine properties that may also help you to calm the effects of the bacterial infection and boost your immunity.

You can always utilize the aloe Vera as a proper treatment procedure on how to treat bacterial infection by applying all the gel on the affected part of the skin. You should leave it for few minutes before rinsing it off with some warm water. Another way that you can try is by consuming aloe Vera juice that may also have the same benefit.

**Garlic**

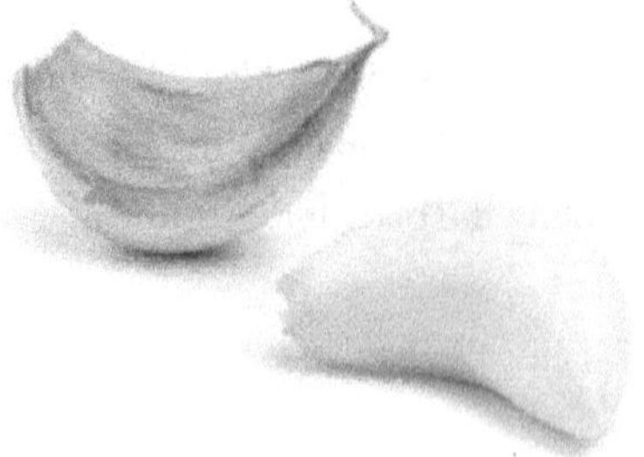

Garlic is available in every kitchen, and it is excellent home remedies to treat a lot of different bacterial and fungal infection. I would also like to suggest that it is a good way to treat bacterial infection by eating at least 4 to 5 cloves of garlic per day.

Moreover, garlic is also considered good for your digestive system. There are multiple yet different ways for you to consume the intake of garlic. You can either chew it or even swallow it. Another way is eating garlic in the form of pharmaceutical capsules.

However, there may be very less and ineffective than directly chewing garlic. Moreover, garlic tea is also another option and recommendation as all the herbal remedy on how to treat and cure your bacterial infection. You would want to add some cloves in the boiling water and steep them some of a few minutes before they are sipping the garlic tea.

Garlic can also be consumed in many ways. The best way is, however, to chew garlic and swallow them raw.

Capsules are widely available as well, even though they might not be as effective. Garlic tea can also help to prepared from boiling some few cloves of garlic and steeping it for at least ten minutes.

**Valerian**

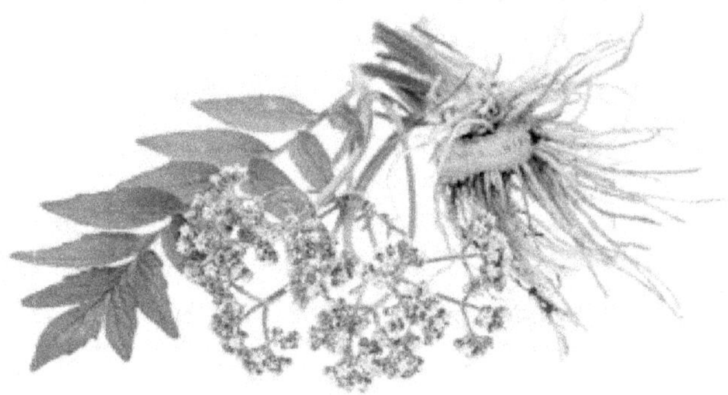

Valerian is also another very popular nighttime home remedies to deal with your anxiety. It contains some elements of mild tranquilizing properties that will almost guarantee you and will get you a good night sleep. However, without all dreaded and the weird hangover feeling early in the morning that you may sometimes have to get with some other pharmaceuticals.

**Passionflower**

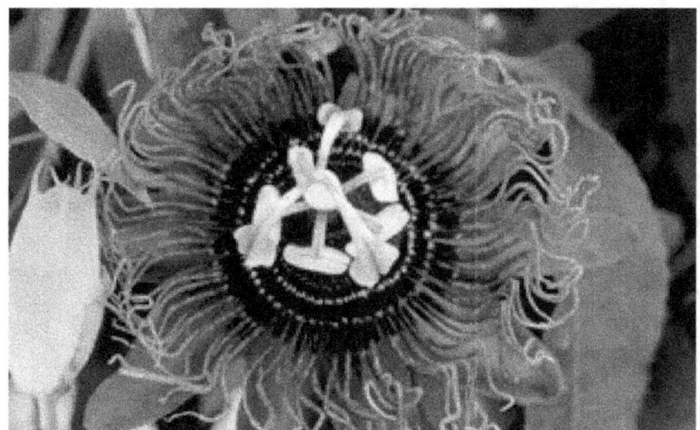

Passionflower is also referred to as folk for a natural remedy and anxiety, insomnia and panic attacks. Passionflower has been shown in many studies to treat anxiety is a very remarkably well.

One study has found it has to be as effective as benzodiazepine drugs, but the only difference is without the drowsiness. Passionflower may also help you to feel an emotionally balanced and exceptionally beneficial way.

Nonetheless, if you suffer from exaggerated emotions then this is by far one of the most efficient home remedies to deal with anxiety, and it needs to be part of your daily regimen.

**Lemon Balm**

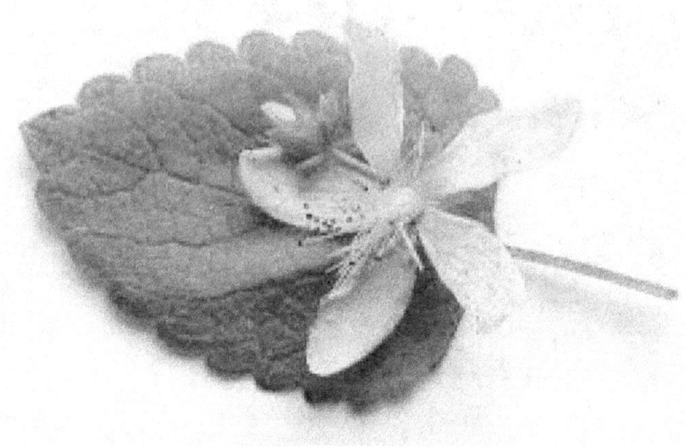

Lemon Balm also is known as 'Melissa officinalis' which is one herbal supplement and tea to treat anxiety and calm your nerves. Some studies suggested that the use of lemon balm can decrease insomnia, anxiety, hyper excitation and fatigue.

A lemon balm extract which should be taken 300mg at breakfast and 300mg at dinner too which may help reduced insomnia mainly due to a decrease in nervousness and also to decreased agitation, guilt, hyperexcitation and fatigue too.

**California poppy**

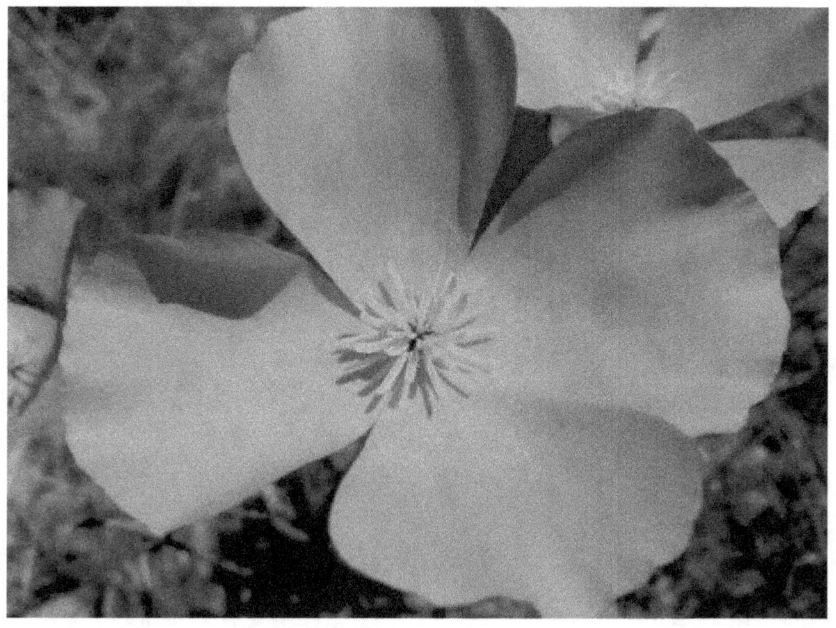

California poppy also called Eschscholtzia californica, which is a tension-relieving, anti-anxiety, sedative, and antispasmodic herb. California poppy also helps with sleeplessness and quells a headache as well as muscular spasm from stress. Some gentle and non-addictive actions are much safer for children and the elderly.


**Wild Lettuce**

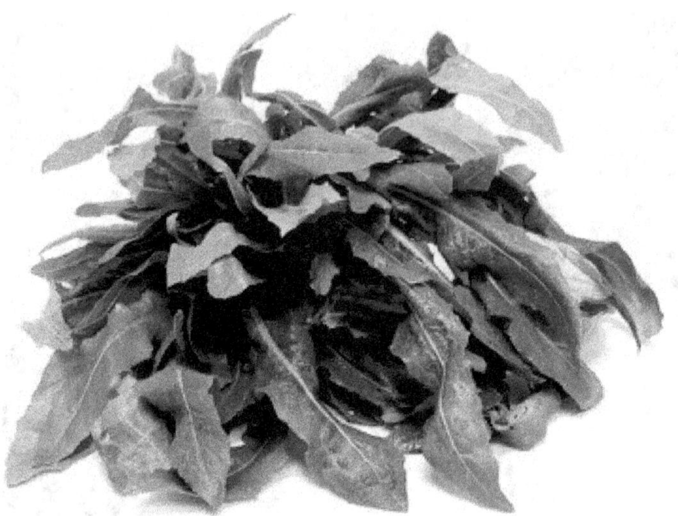

Wild Lettuce is of the species of lactic vireos, which is a mild tranquilizer that may be used for calming a nervous or overactive nervous system. It is very suitable for anxious children or even adolescents. It majorly helps with insomnia. It is also a general pain reliever and antispasmodic that can primarily be used for short coughs.

## Chapter 2 – Herbal Remedies to Treat Your Skin Problems

There are some remedies that prove helpful to treat your irritated and itchy skin. You can treat acne problems and lots of other skin problems. There are some remedies for your assistance.

**Recipe 01: Treatment of Itching with Clay**

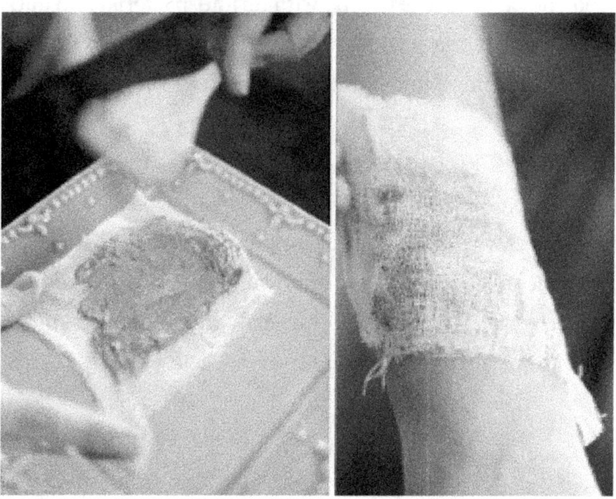

Clay is good for the treatment of itching, acne and various other issues related to your skin. If you want to use clay, mix one cup clay in a bowl and mix it with a small quantity of filtered water to make a creamy paste. Dab your itchy areas with this clay paste and let it dry.

**Clay Pack**

Spread your clay paste on one piece of clean fabric (cotton, muslin, wool and flannel). Put this clay cloth on irritated area so that the clay should directly touch your skin. A bandage wrap or tape can be used to fix this clay patch on your skin for almost four hours.

## Recipe 02: Apple Cider and Clay Recipe

Apple cider can be a good choice to relieve itching with its anti-bacterial and anti-fungal properties. You can use this treatment for dandruff and sunburns. You can directly apply apple vinegar on your skin by putting some drops on washcloth or cotton ball.

If you want to make a clay pack with vinegar, you can substitute water with apple vinegar and make a smooth mixture. You can mix well until you get desired consistency. Apply this paste on a bandage and put clay area on your skin for almost four hours. You can replicate this treatment twice a week.

## Recipe 03: Aloe Vera

This natural herb is excellent to treat you skin problems, such as sunburn, irritation and swelling. Aloe Vera is easy to find in your yard or you can grow it easily.

**Procedure to Use**

You can break off leaves from its plant and cut to open lengthwise from the bottom and top with the help of a knife. Scoop all gooey gel out and carefully rub it on your affected skin and leave it for almost 15 minutes. You can do it on a regular basis until cured. Left over gel can be secured in one airtight container for almost one week.

The rheumatoid arthritis is related to the immune system, and become the reason of inflammation of joints and tissues. The immune system can disturb your overall healthy tissues and organs. You can apply the aloe vera gel to your joint to treat arthritis:

- If you want to get the best results, directly take the plants. It will help you to relieve pain and swelling linked with the rheumatoid arthritis. Cut the leaf from an aloe vera plant with the help of a sharp scissor, and peel its outer leaf to get the gel. You can use your fingers to get the gel out from the plant. Spread the gel on the affected parts just like a lotion, and massage these parts.

- You can also drink the aloe vera juice for the treatment of arthritis. Start your treatment with the small dose that can be 2 to 3 ounces once in a day. You can increase this quantity up to 3 times per day. It will help you to take care of the tenderness in your body, as well as the digestive system.

- You can use aloe vera treatment with other remedies as well because the aloe vera is not only sufficient to treat the rheumatoid arthritis.

**Recipe 04: Oatmeal Remedy**

The oatmeal is one of the greatest remedies for alleviating all skin problems and inflammation because it has a comforting and anti-inflammatory property present in it. It is considered good for the treatment of rashes that may be caused by eczema, poison ivy, sunburn, allergies and chicken pox.

**Procedure to Use:**

To use oatmeal, grind the oatmeal in food processor, blender or coffee crusher. You can mix the ground oatmeal in lukewarm water and put this mixture aside for almost 20 minutes. Apply this mixture on your affected area on a regular basis.

On the other hand, mix ½ cup oatmeal and one-quarter cup powder milk along with honey (2 tablespoons). You can put this blend in one muslin cloth and strongly tie this cloth with the help of a string, rubber band or ribbon, and put in the warm water. Immerse in a great milky bathwater for around 15 minutes. You can pat your skin dry and properly moisturize your affected skin.

For a rash that appears your face, smear thick paste with parallel amount of plain yogurt and oatmeal and mix with some honey. You should leave this mixture on your skin for almost ½ hour and then use lukewarm water to wash it off. Repeat this as much as you can for improved results.

## Recipe 05: Baking Soda

The baking soad always proves good to treat rashes of your skin. It has ability to relieve itching and the inflammation that is associated with rashes.

## Procedure to Use Baking Soda

To work with baking soda, you should take one part of baking soda and mix it with three parts of water. Apply this mixture on particular area of your skin and wait for five minutes before washing your face. You can practice this almost twice in one day and see the improvement.

It is easy to mix some baking soda and coconut oil to make a smooth paste and apply this paste on your rashes. Leave this paste on your skin for almost five minutes and wash your wash. Replicate this procedure twice a day and see improvements.

## Chapter 3 – Herbal Remedies for Insomnia and Anxiety

There are a few treatments that prove helpful for you for anxiety and insomnia. These herbs are really beneficial for everyone.

### Recipe 06: Valerian Root

Valerian is a herb, and its roots are used to make medicine for sleep disorders. It is a common herb used with the combination of hops and lemon balms. The valerian root can cause drowsiness and is ideal for those suffering from the insomnia.

If you are using sleeping pills, then you are advised to treat it with valerian root. There are some scientific evidences that the valerian works for the treatment of sleep disorders. It can also help you to treat the conditions connected with the anxiety and psychological stress that may be asthma, excitants, migraine, headache, upset stomach, etc. It can also be used for the treatment of depression, epilepsy, mild tremors and chronic fatigue.

The women suffering from the menstrual cramps and symptoms of menopause, they can use this herb for their treatment. The extracts and oil of the valerian root are used to flavor different food items and beverages.

## How does it work?

The valerian works like a tranquilizer on your brain and nervous system. Its continuous use will help you to get rid of sleeping pills. It will improve your sleep quality, and bring lots of other benefits with it.

## Side Effects

The Valerian is quite safe to use for the people using it for the medicinal purpose. You can use it for almost 4 to 8 weeks on a constant basis for desired results. There are different side effects of valerian noticed by some people are headache, excitability, and uneasiness.

Some people may have sluggish feelings after having it in the night, but these side effects will be temporary. It will be good to gradually reduce the use of valerian before quitting it completely.

## Interactions of Valerian

- If you are taking valerian, then you have to avoid the use of alcohol because alcohol can be the reason of drowsiness and tiredness.

- The alprazolam can also interact with the valerian because taking both of them at the same time can increase its side effects.

- Benzodiazepine is a sedative medicine and it can strongly interact with valerian causing sleepiness. There is no need to take any sleeping pill and valerian at the same time.

**Accurate Dosage of Valerian**

- If you are suffering from insomnia, then you can take valerian by mouth in the following ways:
- 400 to 900 mg valerian should be extracted for two hours of your sleep time, and you can take it for almost 28 days.
- The 120 mg valerian can be combined with 80 mg lemon balm to take for almost 30 days. Its regular dosage will be 3 times a day.
- You can take the combination of 187 mg valerian extract and make a tablet of 41.9 mg to take almost 2 tablets of the similar quantity at the bedtime for almost 28 days.

**Recipe 07: Chamomile**

Chamomile was a traditional medicine used thousands of years ago for the treatment of anxiety and upset stomach. It is still in use because of its amazing properties because it is considered as a safe plant and used to treat stomach ailments and sleeplessness.

The herb is used with the combination of other plants to get lots of health benefits. If you are suffering from heartburn, upset stomach, nausea, and queasiness, then you can use chamomile. It also proves helpful for the sore mouth and cancer. If you have any skin irritation, the chamomile can help you to heal your wounds.

**Dose of Chamomile**

A standard dosage of the chamomile may vary between 400 milligrams and 1,600 milligrams in a day. You can take it in the form of a capsule, or prepare the tea to drink one to four cups a day. You can use flowers of chamomile to prepare the tea bags, and dip the tea bag in a cup of hot water and cover with a lid for almost 5 to 10 minutes. It is a safe drink for you, but you are advised to let it cool down before drinking it. You can add chamomile flavor for your food items and drinks.

**Side Effects of Chamomile**

Some experts suggested that the chamomile is quite safe to use, but its large doses can cause vomiting. It can also trigger some allergic reactions to the people suffering from relevant allergies with the plants of a daisy family.

- If you are using skin creams of chamomile, you should consider your typical allergic reactions because the chamomile can cause irritation to eyes and eczema.

- You are advised to consult your doctor before taking chamomile because it has a minute amount of coumarin that may affect the thinness of your blood. In some cases, the chamomile is taken before surgery to make your blood thinner, but don't forget to consider its interactions with the anesthetic drugs.

**Interactions of Chamomile**

- If you are taking any drug on a regular basis, such as aspirin, antiplatelet, NSAID painkillers, naproxen, ibuprofen and any other related drugs; you have to consult your doctor before taking chamomile supplements.
- The chamomile can interact with ginkgo Biloba, saw palmetto, valerian, and garlic. It is not advised to take it with any of these herbs.
- The chamomile is not good for pregnant and breastfeeding women. You have to take expert advice before giving it to infants and children.

**Recipe 08: Passionflower**

The above part of the passionflower plant is used to make medicine for the sleep problems, anxiety, gastrointestinal ailments, nervousness and withdrawal symptoms of the narcotic drugs. It is equally beneficial for the asthma, hysteria, seizures, nervousness, irregular heartbeat and high blood pressure.

It can also be used to treat skin burns, pains and swelling. Its extracts are used in the food and beverages to flavor them. It can be used with the combination of other drugs to prop up tranquility and relaxation.

You can combine it with the hops, skullcap, kava, valerian and German chamomile. The chemicals found in the passionflower can make you calm and promote good sleep by relieving the effects of muscle spasm.

**Side Effects of Passionflower**

- The passion flower is found in the food and taken orally to treat insomnia. It should be taken in smaller amounts for the short period of time.
- The passionflower can cause confusion, giddiness, and irregular muscle functions. It may be the reason of inflamed blood vessels.
- You may feel nausea, vomiting, increase in the heart rate and irritations on the skin.
- Interactions of the Passionflower

The passionflower can interact with the narcotic medications because it can cause sleepiness with the use of sedative drugs. It should not be good to use with pentobarbital (Nembutal), Phenobarbital, secobarbital, clonazepam, lorazepam, zolpidem, and other drugs.

**Dose of Passionflower**

If you want to take passionflower by mouth, following are some dosage details for you:

- For the treatment of generalized anxiety disorder, you can take 45 drops of the passion flower liquid on a regular basis.
- A 90 mg tablet can also be used for the treatment of GAD.
- If you want to reduce the symptoms of narcotic withdrawal, then you can use 60 drops of the passionflower in a liquid with 0.8 mg of clonidine.

## Chapter 4 – Herbs for Common Sickness

There are different plants that will help you to treat blood sugar, arthritis pain, cholesterol and various other conditions. The herbs are used for hundreds of years to kill cancer cells and withdrawal symptoms of alcohol. These are effective because of no side effects, and these are easy on your budget because most of the herbs are already available in your kitchen. You can try your own recipe to get the benefits of the natural herbs.

For your convenience, following are some natural herbs that are safe to use, and you can enjoy their health benefits without any stress:

### Recipe 09: Ginger

The ginger is a perfect herbal antibiotic to avoid nausea because it can treat an upset stomach. It can be used during pregnancy, motion disease, and chemotherapy.

The ginger serves as a powerful antioxidant and can block the effects of serotonin. The serotonin is a chemical produced by the stomach and brain. It is quite effective to use in the motion sickness as compared to any traditional drug. It is an effective natural antibiotic to reduce blood pressure, melanoma and arthritis sting.

### Dose of Ginger

- If you want to treat nausea with ginger, instantly take it before the start of symptoms. You may take it 30 minutes before leaving.
- Capsules of ginger are available; you can take almost 500 to 1,000 mg dried ginger in every four hours to treat nausea. The treatment will be continued for the 48 days.

## Recipe 10: Garlic

The garlic contains volatile oils and the particular odor of the garlic has an antibiotic quality because of its allicin contents. It can be included in the regular food or eat it as a medicine. If you are suffering from cough, cold, flow and digestive problem, you can use garlic.

## Dose of Garlic

If you want to maximize the benefits of garlic, you can use the fresh garlic in a crushed form. It is perfect to fight with cancer and cardiovascular diseases. If you want to treat your blood pressure, you can use 5 cloves of garlic in a day. The garlic is also available in a capsule form, try 1,000 mg of garlic extracts in capsule forms.

## Recipe 11: Licorice Root

The licorice is a plant and its roots are used to make medicine. It is used to flavor foods, beverages, and tobacco. If you are suffering from digestive system problems, then you can use it because it is perfect to treat colic, stomach ulcers, and heartburn. It is also beneficial to use for constant gastritis. It is also useful for the infections of bacteria, including cough, bronchitis, and sore throat.

You can use it for liver disorders, malaria, CFS (chronic fatigue syndrome), food poisoning and tuberculosis. It can be used with the combination of Panax ginseng and Bupleurum falciparum to enhance its benefits. It is important to produce essential hormones that enable your body to response stress.

If you want to increase the fertility of women, then the licorice can be used with another herb known as shakuyaku-kanzo-to. It helps in the treatment of the polycystic ovary syndrome. Sometimes, it is used to treat the oily hair, and it contains several chemicals to decrease the swelling and cough. It can make the mucus secretions thin, and enhance the chemicals in the body requires treating ulcers.

**Side Effects of Licorice**

- The licorice is used for food and medicinal purposes in larger amounts. Its purpose is to treat different ailments in a short period of time. It can be applied to the skin for a short period of time to heal it.

- It is unsafe to use more than 4 weeks because the long-term consumption of the licorice can be the reason of high blood pressure, paralysis, low potassium levels, brain damage and heart disease. It should not be consumed on a frequent basis to avoid these side effects.

**Interactions of the Licorice**

The licorice can interact with warfarin because the warfarin is typically used to reduce the blood clotting. The body usually works to break down the warfarin to expel it out from your body. The licorice can increase the breakdown process and reduce its efficiency. You have to check your blood on a regular basis to check the dosage of warfarin.

## Dosage of Licorice

If you want to treat an upset stomach, you can treat it with the particular combination of licorice and different other herbs. Take 1 mL three times a day to get its maximum benefits.

## Chapter 5 – Herbal Remedies for Digestive and Urinary Problems

There are some remedies that prove helpful to treat urinary and digestive problems. These remedies prove helpful for everyone:

### Recipe 12: Cat's Claw

The Cat's claw is a useful herb to treat stomach problem. It is famous for its exceptional properties to strengthen the immune system of your body. It will enable your body to fight infections and different infections. The oxindole alkaloids can enhance the capacity of the immune system to destroy the pathogens. You can use this herb for the treatment painful and swollen joints, and the 8 weeks are enough to treat different health problems.

### Dosage of the Cat's Claw

- You can take one gram of root bark 2 to 3 times a day, and the ideal dosage of the root is 20 to 30 mg. You should not take the products of the cat's claw before surgery and immunosuppressant therapy.

- There can be some adverse reactions of the herb, including stomach pain, diarrhea, and nausea. If you want to avoid the side effects of this herb, then you should take its limited dose. Consult your doctor to know either herb can interact with your current medication.

### Recipe 13: Turmeric

Turmeric is a very powerful herb, which is labeled even to reduce and treat many other cancerous tumors. The Curcumin or Turmeric, which is present in turmeric, has many antibacterial and anti-inflammatory properties along with some high antioxidant content.

## Procedure to Use

Turmeric paste can be made from any sorts of freshly ground turmeric that can always be is applied on the skin for multiple bacterial skin infections.

Turmeric powder can also be consumed along with a glass of warm milk or even water for any respiratory infections. Turmeric can also be used as a secure and a preventive element for many other bacterial infections and of the body by adding it by plenty of nutrition in your diet or even taking curcumin supplements or some teaspoon of turmeric every day.

## Recipe 14: Cabbage

The cabbage is an important member of the cruciferous family of vegetables, including cauliflower, kale, broccoli and sprouts. The cabbage is famous for its healing power because the sulfur compounds in the cabbage are ideal to treat cancer. It is high in vitamin C, and one cup of cabbage may serve as a natural antibiotic.

## Procedure to Use Cabbage

A cup of fresh cabbage juice 2 to 3 times a day will help you to treat stomach ulcers. You can add a half teaspoon of honey in the cabbage juice to enhance its taste. You can chew raw cabbage to get its enzymes. The leaves of raw cabbage may help you to treat tender breasts and inflammation caused by the mastitis and fibro cysts.

## Recipe 15: Garlic

If you want to look for ways on how to some treat bacterial infection, then you should not skip any ginger effect, which is very efficient in treating factors like stomach infection and other respiratory disease.

## Procedure to Use Garlic

It helps to cool down your body and boost your blood circulation at the same time. As a result, the ginger effect will help you to reduce the amount of all the bad bacteria in your body. To treat and cure your respiratory infection, it is also highly recommended that you are drinking ginger at least tea 3-4 times during a day.

Moreover, you can always massage your affected skin by garlic pieces. By boosting all the blood circulation, this is the way we will help you reduce the pain that is caused by bacterial infection.

Ginger extract can always be used for the massaging on the affected areas of the body for the treating bacterial infections and for controlling all the pain. For instance, take a stalk of ginger on every day to prevent infections of all the body.

## Conclusion

People are turning to natural remedies aka home remedies, or natural cures, for their ailments or other diseases because these treatments are entirely made with natural ingredients such as fruits, herbs, and vegetables. All ingredients that maybe readily found at home are the reason why people prefer natural remedies. Home remedies do not always promote the use of harsh chemicals that are inexpensive and usually do not produce any side effects, whatsoever. People also enjoy making something very useful to use instead of paying some expensive over-the-counter drugs that can have very dangerous side effects.

Humans throughout the history have relied on natural remedies before the invention of modern medicine and other synthetic drugs. Most common ailments have known to be treatments with ingredients that are found in your kitchen. Researchers have also discovered that thousands of healing nutrients in the foods are those that we eat every day.

Therefore, through this book, an attempt has been made to help create awareness among people about the brilliant use of natural remedies that could help in every way possible and cure all the deadly and the routine based diseases, viruses, and infections.